Coconut: Detox Diet:

Gluten Free Recipes for Celiac Disease, Wheat Free & Paleo Free; Detox Cleanse Diet to Lose Belly Fat & Increase Energy

Emma Rose

Coconut Flour Recipes for Optimal Health and Quick Weight Loss

Gluten Free Recipes for Celiac Disease, Gluten Sensitivities, and Paleo Free Diets

Emma Rose

Table of Contents

Introduction

I want to thank you and congratulate you for purchasing the book, *"**Coconut Flour Recipes for Optimal Health and Quick Weight Loss**: Gluten Free Recipes for Celiac Disease, Gluten Sensitivities, and Paleo Free Diets"*.

This book contains proven steps and strategies on how to integrate coconut flour into your diet for a healthier food lifestyle.

In this book, you will learn about the benefits of using coconut flour and how it can help you lose weight and become healthier without limiting the food you're eating. I have also included several guilt-free coconut flour recipes that you and your loved ones will surely enjoy.

Thanks again for purchasing this book, I hope you enjoy it! Please take some time to stop by and LIKE our Facebook page:

https://www.facebook.com/joypublishing

With gratitude,

Emma Rose

Chapter 1: Why Use Coconut Flour?

Nowadays, people are getting more conscious about their food lifestyle and how it affects their overall well-being. Most of the foods that are available today are processed or refined however there are some good alternatives that can be used without taking away much from flavor.

Among the healthy alternatives for refined grains is the coconut flour. Coconut flour is one of the best alternatives to replace the usual refined wheat flour. Since coconut flour is very versatile, it can be used to replace refined grains from almost all kinds of baked goods and meals.

There are five major advantages in using coconut flour:

1. Coconut flour is gluten free. For people who have allergies or are sensitive to gluten, coconut flour is definitely a gift from heaven. By using coconut flour, people allergic to gluten will be able to enjoy baked treats.

2. Coconut flour improves cell regeneration. This type of flour has high non-gluten protein content that helps improve the growth of cells and rejuvenation.

3. Coconut flour is high in fiber. For people who want to lose or maintain their weight, coconut flour is a good alternative ingredient to make your own breads and cakes without feeling guilty about it. Foods made with coconut flour makes a person feel fuller faster and longer.

4. Coconut flour has high manganese content which means this ingredient will enable you to absorb more nutrients from foods faster. Also, manganese is proven to promote healthy blood sugar levels and thyroid health.

5. Coconut flour contains lauric acid. This healthy saturated fat is important to a person's immune health and it promotes healthy skin.

Though coconut flour can be used as a substitute ingredient to almost all recipes calling for wheat flour, it also takes some tweaking with the other ingredients for it to work well with baking and cooking. For example, coconut flour is drier than wheat flour therefore it requires more water when used in baking. The following are recipes that you can use to start your journey to a healthier you.

Chapter 2: Coconut Flour Bread Recipes

Zucchini Bread

Ingredients:

- ½ cup of coconut flour

- ¾ tsp of baking soda

- ½ tsp of salt

- 1 tbsp of cinnamon

- ½ tsp of nutmeg

- 4 pcs of pasture-raised eggs

- 3 tbsp of raw honey OR grade B maple syrup

- 1 cup of zucchini, shred it finely

- 1 pc of ripe banana, mashed

- 1 tbsp of coconut oil

- ½ cup of walnuts

Procedure:

1. Turn on the oven and set it to 350F.

2. Prepare a loaf pan and grease it with coconut oil. You can also line the pan with parchment paper, if available. Set the pan aside.

3. Prepare a piece of cheesecloth or a nut milk bag and place the finely shredded zucchini inside. Squeeze as hard as you can to remove the excess moisture from the zucchini.

4. In a large mixing bowl, combine the egg, honey or maple syrup, and banana. Mix together until the ingredients are well-incorporated.

5. Add in the coconut flour, baking soda, salt, cinnamon, and nutmeg into the mixing bowl and mix well. Then, add in the shredded zucchini and stir until the mixture becomes smooth.

6. Add in the walnuts and stir.

7. Pour the batter into the loaf pan and place it inside the oven. Bake for 45 to 50 minutes or until the bread has completely set.

Coco Doughnuts

Ingredients:

- ½ cup of coconut flour

- ¼ tsp of sea salt

- ¼ tsp of baking soda

- 6 pcs of eggs

- ½ cup of honey

- 1 tbsp of vanilla

- ½ cup of unsalted butter OR coconut oil, already melted

- 5 tbsp of honey

- Coconut flakes for toppings

Procedure:

1. Turn on the oven and set it to 350F.

2. In a mixing bowl, combine the coconut flour, sea salt, and baking soda. Stir the dry ingredients together until well-mixed.

3. Add in the eggs, honey, vanilla, and butter into the mixing bowl. Use a whisk or a hand mixer set on low to blend all of the ingredients together.

4. Prepare about 8 donut pan circles and fill each pan with the batter about 2/3 of the way.

5. Place the donut pan circles into the oven and bake for 20 minutes.

6. While baking, warm 5 tablespoons of honey and place it in a saucer. Then, toast the coconut flakes.

7. Dip each piece of donut in the honey and sprinkle it with the toasted coconut flakes.

Coco Bread

Ingredients:

- ¾ cup of coconut flour

- 1 tsp of baking soda

- A pinch of sea salt

- 4 pcs of whole eggs

- 3 pcs of eggs, white and yolk separated

- 5 tbsp of organic butter

- 3 tbsp of coconut milk

- 1 tbsp of raw honey

- Organic virgin coconut oil

Procedure:

1. Prepare a loaf pan and lightly grease it using the coconut oil. Then, line the loaf pan with baking paper with a coating of coconut oil just to make sure that the loaf does not stick to the pan.

2. Turn on the oven and set it to 350F.

3. Take the egg whites from three eggs and whisk it until it become stiff. You can use a hand mixer if you like. Set it aside.

4. Take the egg yolks and pour it in a food processor. Add in the four whole eggs, organic butter, coconut milk, and raw honey. Blend the ingredients until thoroughly combined.

5. Add in the coconut flour, baking soda, and salt gradually into the food processor while blending. Continue to process the ingredients until the mixture becomes thick in consistency.

6. Prepare a large mixing bowl and pour in the mixture from the food processor. Take the egg whites and fold it in the mixture.

7. Once the mixture and egg whites are thoroughly combined, pour in the batter into the loaf pan. Place the pan inside the oven and bake for 40 minutes.

8. Reduce the heat to 300F and cover the loaf pan. Cook for another 5 to 10 minutes.

9. Once cooked, remove the loaf pan from the oven and place it on a cooling rack to cool completely before slicing and serving.

Chocolate Muffin

Ingredients:

- ½ cup of coconut flour

- 1 tsp of baking soda

- A dash of salt

- ¼ cup of coconut sugar

- 2 tbsp of cocoa powder

- 1 tsp of vanilla extract

- ¼ cup of coconut oil

- 2/3 cup of coconut milk

- 4 pcs of pastured eggs

- 1 tsp of apple cider vinegar

Procedure:

1. Turn on the oven and set it to 350F.

2. Melt the coconut oil and place it in a bowl or a food processor. Add in the coconut flour, baking soda, salt, coconut sugar, cocoa powder, vanilla extract, coconut milk, eggs, and apple cider vinegar. Stir or blend the ingredients together until it forms a smooth batter.

3. Prepare a muffin tin and line it with paper or silicone liners.

4. Pour the batter about ¾ of the way of each muffin liner as the muffin will rise once it is cooked.

5. Place the muffin tin inside the oven and bake for 20 to 30 minutes.

Cheese Biscuits

Ingredients:

- 1/3 cup of coconut flour
- ¼ cup of butter, melted
- 4 pcs of eggs
- ¼ tsp of salt
- ¼ tsp of cream of tartar
- 1/8 tsp of baking soda
- ½ cup of shredded cheddar cheese
- ¼ cup of shredded parmesan cheese

Procedure:

1. Turn on the oven and set it to 400F.

2. In a mixing bowl, combine the coconut flour, salt, cream of tartar, and baking soda. Stir and make a well in the center of the dry ingredients.

3. Add in the eggs and melted butter in the center of the dry ingredients and mix. Whisk the ingredients together until it forms a smooth batter.

4. Add in the cheeses and stir to properly combine.

5. Prepare a baking sheet and spray it with cooking spray. Drop spoonfuls of batter into the sheet at even intervals.

6. Place the baking sheet inside the oven and bake for 8 to 10 minutes. Once cooked, let it cool on a wire rack then remove the biscuits from the baking sheet.

Gingerbread Doughnuts

Ingredients:

- 4 pcs of large eggs

- ¼ cup of melted coconut oil

- 1/3 cup of coconut palm sugar

- ¼ cup of full fat coconut milk

- 2 tbsp of blackstrap molasses (unsulphured)

- 1 tsp of raw apple cider vinegar

- 1 ½ tsp of pure vanilla extract

- 1 ¾ tsp of ground cinnamon

- 1 ¼ tsp of ground ginger

- 1 tsp of ground cloves

- ¾ tsp of allspice

- ½ tsp of baking soda

- ¼ tsp of freshly ground nutmeg

- ¼ tsp of sea salt

- 1/8 tsp of cayenne pepper

- ½ cup of coconut flour, sifted

- ½ cup of organic powdered sugar

- 2 tbsp of full fat canned coconut milk

- ¼ tsp of pure vanilla extract

- A pinch of sea salt

Procedure:

1. In a mixing bowl, combine the eggs, melted coconut oil, and palm sugar. Use a hand mixer to beat the ingredients together.

2. In a small bowl, combine the coconut milk, apple cider vinegar, molasses, and vanilla extract. Stir the ingredients together until properly combined. Pour the mixture into the large mixing bowl and beat until the ingredients are well mixed.

3. In a separate small bowl, combine the ground ginger, ground cloves, ground cinnamon, allspice, nutmeg, baking soda, cayenne pepper, and sea salt. Stir the ingredients together. Add in the spice mixture into the mixing bowl and stir until all the ingredients are just combined.

4. Add in the sifted coconut flour into the mixing bowl and use the hand mixer to incorporate all the ingredients. Blend until it forms a smooth batter.

5. Turn on the oven and set it to 350F.

6. Pour the batter into a doughnut pan and place it inside the oven. Bake for 18 to 20 minutes then place it immediately on a cooling rack.

7. While waiting for the doughnuts to cool, prepare a large mixing bowl and combine the organic powdered sugar, coconut milk, vanilla, and salt. Whisk the ingredients together until no lumps are present.

8. Use a spoon to drizzle the glaze over the doughnuts.

Lemon Bread with Lemon Glaze

Ingredients:

- 6 pcs of eggs

- ¼ cup of coconut oil, melted

- Zest of 2 pcs of lemons

- Juice from 2 lemons combined with coconut milk to make 1 cup

- 1/3 cup of honey

- 2/3 cup of coconut flour

- 1 tsp of baking soda

- ¼ tsp of salt

- 2 tbsp of coconut oil

- 2 tbsp of honey

- 2 tbsp of coconut milk

- Zest and juice of 1 lemon

- ½ tsp of vanilla extract

Procedure:

1. Turn on the oven and set it to 350F.

2. In a large mixing bowl, add in the eggs, ¼ cup of coconut oil, zest from 2 pieces of lemons, 1 cup of the lemon juice and coconut milk mixture, 1/3 up of honey, coconut flour, baking soda, and salt. Whisk the ingredients together until it forms a smooth batter.

3. Prepare a loaf pan and grease it with coconut oil. Pour the batter into the pan and place it inside the oven. Bake for 32 to 45 minutes then remove from the oven and set it aside to cool completely.

4. In a small bowl, combine the 2 tablespoons of coconut oil, 2 tablespoons of honey, 2 tbsp of coconut milk, zest and juice of 1 lemon, and vanilla extract. Whisk together until well-incorporated then pour the glaze on top of the loaf.

5. Place the loaf inside the refrigerator for about 30 minutes to help the glaze set before serving.

Chapter 3: Coconut Flour Breakfast Recipes

Coconut Porridge

Ingredients:

- ½ cup of full-fat canned coconut milk

- ¼ cup of water

- 3 tbsp of coconut flour

- 2 tbsp of finely shredded coconut

- ½ of a banana, mashed

- Frozen berries or chopped nuts, will be used for toppings

Procedure:

1. Prepare a small saucepan and add in the coconut milk, water, coconut flour, and the finely shredded coconut. Stir the mixture and let it boil.

2. Place a lid and reduce the heat. Let it simmer for 2 to 3 minutes stirring occasionally.

3. Remove the saucepan from the heat and add in the mashed banana. Whisk to combine and stir.

4. Replace the saucepan into the stove and cook for another 2 minutes. Continue stirring until it thickens.

Coconut Bake

Ingredients:

- 6 tbsp of coconut flour

- 10 pcs of eggs

- 2 tsp of vanilla extract

- 4 pcs of ripe bananas, mashed

- ¼ tsp of salt

Procedure:

1. In a mixing bowl, add in the coconut flour, eggs, vanilla extract, mashed bananas, and salt. Mix the ingredients thoroughly and let it sit for 10 minutes.

2. Prepare a muffin tin by lining it with muffin liners. Then, pour the batter into the tin.

3. Place the muffin tin inside the oven and bake for 20 to 25 minutes at 350F. You can also bake this in your microwave for 3 minutes on high settings. Just remember to use ramekins instead of muffin tins.

Bacon Pancakes

Ingredients:

- 16 pcs of cooked bacon strips

- ¼ cup of mashed ripe banana

- 4 pcs of large eggs

- 6 tbsp of full fat canned coconut milk

- 1 tsp of apple cider vinegar

- 1 tsp of vanilla extract

- 3 tbsp of organic coconut flour

- 1 tsp of cinnamon

- ½ tsp of baking soda

- A pinch of salt

- Coconut oil

- 2 tbsp of maple syrup

Procedure:

1. Place the bacon on a wire rack and bake it in the oven for 10 to 20 minutes at 400F.

2. In a medium mixing bowl, combine the mashed banana, eggs, apple cider vinegar, coconut milk, and vanilla. Whisk the ingredients together until properly combined.

3. In a separate mixing bowl, combine the organic coconut flour, baking soda, cinnamon, and salt. Give it a stir until the ingredients are incorporated.

4. Pour in the banana mixture into the coconut flour mixture and whisk together until the batter has no lumps.

5. Prepare a skillet and heat the coconut oil. Once the oil is hot, add in three tablespoons of batter into the pan. Make a rectangular shaped pancake about the size of your bacon. Flip the pancake once bubbles form on top.

6. Repeat the process until all the batter is cooked then assemble the pancakes. Place strips of bacon on top of a pancake then drizzle with a bit of maple syrup. Put another pancake on top and enjoy.

Strawberry Flapjacks

Ingredients:

- 1 pc of egg

- 1 tbsp of almond flour

- 1 tsp of coconut flour

- Coconut oil

- ¼ tsp of baking soda

- ½ tsp of cream of tartar

- Stevia

- Organic strawberries

Procedure:

1. Prepare a skillet and heat the coconut oil.

2. In a small bowl, whisk the egg and adding in a splash of water. Once combined, add in the almond flour and coconut flour and whisk again.

3. Add in the baking soda, stevia, and cream of tartar. Mix the ingredients together until it forms a smooth batter. You can taste the batter to gauge the amount of stevia needed.

4. Slice the strawberries into thin slices.

5. Pour the batter into the pan to make one mini-pancake. Once the pancake is slightly firm, place strawberry slices on top. Flip the pancake to cook the other side.

Oats and Flax Crisps

Ingredients:

- 2/3 cup of rolled oats

- 1/3 cup of flax seeds

- ½ cup of shredded coconut

- ¼ cup of coconut oil, melted

- 1/3 cup of unsweetened coconut milk

- 3 tbsp of maple syrup

- 2 tbsp of coconut flour

- 1 tbsp of coconut sugar

- 1 tbsp of chia seeds

- 3 tsp of ground ginger

- 1 tsp of cinnamon

- 1 tsp of pure vanilla extract

- ¼ tsp of salt

Procedure:

1. Turn on the oven and set it to 350F. Prepare two baking sheets and line it with silicone mats or parchment paper.

2. In a large mixing bowl, combine the rolled oats, flax seeds, shredded coconut, coconut flour, coconut sugar, chia seeds, ground ginger, cinnamon, and salt. Stir the ingredients together until evenly combined.

3. In a separate bowl, combine the coconut oil, coconut milk, maple syrup, and vanilla extract. Stir the ingredients until well-mixed. Then, pour the mixture over the dry ingredients. Stir the ingredients together until properly incorporated.

4. Drop a spoonful of the mixture into the baking sheets and flatten it with the back of the spoon to make thin biscuit-like crisps.

5. Place the baking sheets in the oven and bake for 18 to 25 minutes. Once cooked, remove the baking sheets from the oven and set it aside to cool completely.

Chapter 4: Coconut Flour Cake Recipes

Apple and Cinnamon Cake

Ingredients:

- 6 pcs of free-range eggs

- 1 cup of coconut oil OR organic butter, already melted

- ¼ cup of raw honey

- 1 pc of apple, grated

- Zest of 1 pc of lemon

- ½ cup of coconut flour

- 1 cup of desiccated coconut

- 2 tsp of cinnamon

- 1 tsp of baking soda

- A pinch of sea salt

- 1 pc of apple, slice it into very thin wedges

- Juice of ½ of a lemon

- Extra coconut flour for dusting

Procedure:

1. Turn on the oven and set it to 150C.

2. Prepare a cake tin and spray it with cooking oil. You can also line it with parchment paper if you prefer.

3. In a food processor, add in the eggs, coconut oil, honey, grated apple, lemon zest, coconut flour, desiccated coconut, cinnamon, baking soda, and sea salt. Blend all of the ingredients together until properly combined.

4. Spoon the batter into the cake tin and spread it evenly.

5. Arrange the wedges of apples on top of the batter. Decorate it however you like. Then, squeeze the lemon juice on the apples.

6. Place the cake tin inside the oven and bake for 45 minutes.

7. Once cooked, let it cool complete before transferring it into a serving plate. Dust with the extra coconut flour before serving.

Coffee Cake

Ingredients:

- 1 cup of coconut flour

- ½ tsp of Celtic sea salt

- 1 tsp of ground cinnamon

- 8 pcs of large organic eggs

- 1 tsp of baking soda

- ½ cup of strained plain coconut milk yogurt

- 5 tbsp of coconut oil

- ½ cup of honey

- 1 tbsp of vanilla extract

- 1 ½ cups of nuts

- 2 tsp of cinnamon

- 4 tbsp of honey

- 4 tbsp of cold coconut oil, cut it into tablespoons

Procedure:

1. Turn on the oven and set it to 325F. Place the rack in the middle part of the oven.

2. In a food processor, combine the coconut flour, sea salt, 1 teaspoon of ground cinnamon, eggs, baking soda, coconut milk yogurt, 5 tablespoons of coconut oil, ½ cup of honey, and vanilla extract. Blend the ingredients until the mixture becomes smooth.

3. Prepare an 8" x 8" baking dish and pour in the batter inside.

4. Wash and dry the food processor bowl. Add in your choice of nuts, 2 teaspoons of cinnamon, 4 tablespoons of honey, and 4 tablespoons of coconut oil. Process until the nuts are coarsely chopped and all of the ingredients bind together.

5. Spoon the topping on the batter and spread it across the surface of the batter.

6. Place the baking dish in the oven and bake for 40 to 45 minutes. Once cooked, place it on a wire rack and let it cool for about 20 minutes before cutting and serving.

Chocolate Cake

Ingredients:

- ¾ cup of coconut flour, sifted
- ¼ cup of cacao powder
- 1 tsp of Celtic sea salt
- 1 tsp of baking soda
- 10 pcs of eggs
- 1 cup of coconut oil
- 1 ½ cups of coconut sugar
- 1 tbsp of vanilla extract
- ¼ tsp of orange zest
- 1 cup of dark chocolate
- ½ cup of grapeseed oil
- 2 tbsp of agave nectar
- 1 tbsp of vanilla extract
- A pinch of Celtic sea salt

Procedure:

1. In a small mixing bowl, combine the coconut flour, cacao powder, Celtic sea salt, and baking soda. Mix the ingredients together.

2. In a large mixing bowl, combine the eggs, coconut oil, coconut sugar, vanilla extract, and orange zest. Use a hand mixer to mix the ingredients until properly incorporated.

3. Gradually add in the dry ingredients mixture into the large bowl while blending with the hand mixer.

4. Prepare two 9" round cake pans. Lightly grease it with oil and dust using the coconut flour. Pour the batter inside the cake pans and place it inside the oven.

5. Set the oven to 325F and bake for 35 to 40 minutes.

6. Once cooked, remove from the oven and place it on a cooling rack to cool completely.

7. Prepare a small saucepan and add in the dark chocolate and grapeseed oil. Combine the two ingredients over low heat.

8. Add in the agave nectar, vanilla extract, and salt into the saucepan. Stir until the ingredients are well-incorporated.

9. Remove from the heat and place it inside the freezer for about 15 minutes.

10. Once cool, remove the frosting from the freezer and use the hand mixer to whip the frosting until it becomes thick and fluffy.

11. Place the frosting in between the two layers of cakes. Place one cake on top of the other and use the remaining frosting to cover the top of the cake.

Double Chocolate Beet Root Brownies

Ingredients:

- 4 pcs of large pastured eggs

- 1/3 cup of coconut oil, melted

- 1 tsp of vanilla extract

- ¾ cup of maple syrup

- 1 ½ cups of beet puree

- 2 tbsp of coconut cream

- ½ cup of coconut flour

- ½ cup of raw cocoa powder

- ½ tsp of unrefined salt

- ½ tsp of baking soda

- ½ cup of chocolate chips

Procedure:

1. Turn on the oven and set it to 350F.

2. In a large mixing bowl, combine the eggs, coconut oil, vanilla extract, maple syrup, beet puree, and coconut

cream. Use a hand mixer to thoroughly mix the ingredients.

3. In another bowl, combine the coconut flour, cocoa powder, salt, baking soda, and chocolate chips. Stir to mix the ingredients together.

4. Gradually add in the dry ingredients into the large mixing bowl containing the wet ingredients. Use the hand mixer to properly combine the ingredients.

5. Prepare an 8" x 8" baking pan and grease it lightly with coconut oil. Then, pour the batter into the pan.

6. Place the baking pan inside the oven and bake for 35 to 40 minutes.

Pumpkin Bars

Ingredients:

- 1 ½ cups of pumpkin puree

- ¾ cup of coconut flour

- ¾ cup of maple syrup

- 1 ½ tsp of ground cinnamon

- ¾ tsp of ground ginger

- ¼ tsp of ground cloves

- ¾ tsp of baking soda

- ¼ tsp of salt

- 2 pcs of large eggs

- Coconut oil

Procedure:

1. Turn on the oven and set it to 350F.

2. Prepare a 9" x 9" baking dish and lightly grease it using the coconut oil.

3. In a large mixing bowl, combine the pumpkin puree, coconut flour, maple syrup, ground cinnamon, ground

cloves, ground ginger, baking soda, salt, and eggs. Stir the ingredients together until well-incorporated.

4. Pour the batter into the baking dish and smooth the top. Place the baking dish inside the oven and bake for 40 to 45 minutes. Once cooked, let it cool completely before cutting and serving.

Chocolate Chip Banana Cookies

Ingredients:

- 1 pc of ripe banana

- 1 pc of large egg

- 2 tbsp of extra virgin coconut oil

- 3 tbsp of coconut flour, sifted

- 1 tbsp of vanilla extract

- ½ tsp of cream of tartar

- 1/8 tsp of baking soda

- 1/8 tsp of sea salt

- ¼ cup of chocolate chips

Procedure:

1. Turn on the oven and set it to 325F.

2. Prepare a baking pan and line it with parchment paper.

3. In a large mixing bowl, combine the banana and egg. Use a hand mixer to mix the ingredients together. Slowly add in the coconut oil while mixing.

4. Add in the coconut flour, vanilla extract, cream of tartar, baking soda, and sea salt. Blend the ingredients until it forms a smooth batter.

5. Add in the chocolate chips into the batter and stir.

6. Use a spoon to drop about 1 inch balls of batter on the baking pan then flatten the batter to form a cookie shape. Leave enough space between each cookie.

7. Place the baking pan inside the oven and bake for 40 minutes.

Classic Vanilla Cake

Ingredients:

- 4 pcs of large eggs, whites and yolks separated

- 1 tsp of cream of tartar

- ¼ cup of extra virgin coconut oil

- 3 tbsp of raw honey

- ¼ cup of coconut flour, sifted

- 2 tsp of vanilla extract

- ¼ tsp of baking soda

- 1/8 tsp of salt

Procedure:

1. Turn on the oven and set it to 350F.

2. Prepare an 8" x 1.5" round cake pan and line it with parchment paper.

3. In a large mixing bowl, combine the cream of tartar with the egg whites. Use a whisk or a hand mixer to whip the ingredients together to form stiff peaks.

4. In a separate mixing bowl, combine the honey and coconut oil. Use a hand mixer to mix the two

44

ingredients to form a cream. Add in the egg yolks, and mix again.

5. Gradually add in the coconut flour, vanilla extract, baking soda, and salt into the mixture. Use the hand mixer to combine the ingredients until it forms a smooth batter.

6. Pour the batter into the bowl with the whipped egg whites and fold until properly incorporated. Pour the mixture into the cake pan.

7. Place the cake pan in the oven and bake for 20 minutes.

Lady Finger Cookies

Ingredients:

- 4 pcs of pastured eggs, separate the white from the yolk

- ¼ cup of maple syrup

- ¼ tsp of baking soda

- ½ tsp of vanilla extract

- 1/3 cup of coconut flour, sifted

- 1 tsp of freshly ground coffee

Procedure:

1. Turn on the oven and set it to 400F.

2. Place the egg whites in a mixing bowl and beat it until stiff peaks form using a hand mixer.

3. In a large mixing bowl, add in the egg yolks, vanilla extract, baking soda, and maple syrup. Whisk the ingredients together until properly combined. Add in the sifted coconut flour and continue to mix the ingredients until it forms a smooth batter.

4. Fold the egg whites into the mixture then add in the ground coffee.

5. Prepare a baking sheet and line it with parchment paper. Pour the batter into a pipe bag and attach a

round pipe tube at the end. Make about 3-in long cookies on the baking sheet.

6. Place the baking sheet inside the oven and bake for 13 minutes. Once down, set it aside to cool completely before serving.

Custard Cake

Ingredients:

- 4 pcs of eggs

- 2 cups of milk

- ½ cup of coconut flour

- ½ cup of raw honey

- 1 tsp of pure vanilla extract

- 2 tsp of baking powder

- ¼ cup of butter, melted

- 1 ½ cups of unsweetened coconut flakes

- ½ cup of chocolate chips

Procedure:

1. Turn on the oven and set it to 350F.

2. In a large bowl, add in the eggs, coconut flour, milk, honey, vanilla extract, baking powder, and butter. Whisk the ingredients together until it forms a smooth batter. You can use a hand mixer if you prefer.

3. Add in the chocolate chips and coconut flakes. Stir until all ingredients are properly combined.

4. Prepare an 8" cake pan and pour the batter inside. Place the pan inside the oven and bake for 45 to 50 minutes.

5. Once cooked, let it rest and cool completely before splicing and serving.

Conclusion

Thank you again for purchasing *"**Coconut Flour Recipes for Optimal Health and Quick Weight Loss**: Gluten Free Recipes for Celiac Disease, Gluten Sensitivities, and Paleo Free Diets"*!

I hope this book was able to help you to discover the benefits of using coconut flour.

The next step is to enjoy the recipes you have learned to make healthier foods for yourself and your loved ones.

Loosing weight and changing your lifestyle isn't easy. We all need motivation to keep our goal in mind.

Finally, if you enjoyed this book, please take the time to share your thoughts and post a review on Amazon. It'd be greatly appreciated!

I would love for you to share your experiences, stories and encouragements with me. My email address is emmarosekindle@gmail.com

With sincere thanks,

Emma Rose

Emma Rose

Preview of "The Almond Flour Recipes for Optimal Health and Quick Weight Loss: Gluten Free Recipes for Celiac Disease, Gluten Sensitivities, and Paleo Free Diets"

Chapter 1: Almond Flour

Almond is native to the northern Indian subcontinent. The almond seed is more of a drupe than a nut. Like peaches, cherries and apricots, almond trees bears fruits with seeds inside which are commonly referred to as almond nut.

Almond flour is a popular substitute to wheat flour in baking and cooking. This is made from whole almonds with the skins removed. This is often preferred by health conscious individuals because it is gluten-free, high in fiber and low in carbohydrates. It is also an excellent source of protein. Almond flour is also rich in vitamins and minerals including magnesium, potassium and vitamin E.

Benefits of using almond flour:

Nutrients

Almond flour contains Vitamin E which can help prevent cell damage and heart disease. It also contains calcium which strengthens the bone and helps your circulatory system carry hormones throughout your body. Almond flour is also rich in potassium which can regulate your blood pressure.

Easy to Prepare

You can purchase almond flour in your local grocery or make it yourself. Just submerge the almonds in boiling water for a minute. Place in a strainer and remove the skin. Allow to dry then place in a coffee grinder or food processor. Process until it becomes very fine.

Complementary Foods

Serving dishes and pasties with almond flour can supplement the protein that you get from meat. It also balances your diet if it is served with fruits and vegetables. Almond flour can also compliment gluten free and low carbohydrate diets.

Reduces Heart Disease Risk

Almond contains high amounts of monounsaturated fats. This is the type of fat found in olive oil which is associated with good heart health. The antioxidants in the almond flour can also help keep the arteries healthy.

Chapter 2: Bread and Pancakes

Paleo Pumpkin Bread

Ingredients:

- 1 cup blanched almond

- ½ tsp baking soda

- 1 tsp nutmeg

- ½ cup roasted pumpkin

- ¼ tsp stevia

- ¼ tsp Celtic sea salt

- 1 tbsp ground cinnamon

- ½ tsp cloves

- 2 tbsp honey

- 3 large eggs

Procedure:

1. Combine the spices such as cinnamon, cloves, nutmeg, and cloves along with the almond flour and salt in a food processor.

2. Blend few times then add the stevia, pumpkin, eggs and honey.

3. Transfer the batter into a loaf pan.

4. Bake for 45 minutes at 350 degrees.

5. Allow to cool for an hour before slicing.

6. Serve alone or with your favorite spread.

Check out the rest of "Almond Flour Recipes for Optimal Health and Quick Weight Loss: Gluten Free Recipes for Celiac Disease, Gluten Sensitivities, and Paleo Free Diets" on Amazon.

Or go to: http://amzn.to/1qx2LaT

Detox Diet Guide

Lose Weight Quickly, Achieve Optimal Health and Feel Energized Through the 10 Day Detox

Emma Rose

Table of Contents

Introduction

I want to thank you and congratulate you for purchasing the book, *"Detox Diet Guide: Lose Weight Quickly, Achieve Optimal Health and Feel Energized Through the 10 Day Detox"*.

This book contains proven steps and strategies on how to not just simply flush out toxic substances from our bodies, but to also enhance the way our bodies naturally flush out those toxins.

It also contains other important information such as the most common toxins that are found in the environment that we unknowingly consume, the many ways our bodies naturally detoxify themselves, the things one must and must not do within the ten days of the detox diet, detoxification recipes that can be easily prepared, and some important reminders that must be taken before, during, and after the detox diet.

Thanks again for purchasing this book. I hope you enjoy it! Please take some time to stop by and LIKE our Facebook page:

https://www.facebook.com/joypublishing

With gratitude,

Emma Rose

Chapter 1: Toxins and the Body

As the human body does its usual processes, some things need to be expelled. These are usually waste products made as a result of filtering out substances not needed by the body. There is a reason for the so-called "calls of nature" – which are peeing and releasing excrement.

But sometimes, those unwanted substances can build up in the organs and the bodily systems that comprise them. If there are too much of those substances, they will cause all sorts of harm to the overall bodily functions that can lead to various ailments.

The Top 10 List of Most Common Toxins

Human civilization evolves as a result of the desire of the people to live more comfortably and conveniently. But in the process of that evolution, it has unknowingly unleashed a cavalcade of impurities that do not just pollute the environment, but also the human body. Despite the many efforts by several government agencies and private individuals to thwart the sources of those impurities, there are traces of those impurities that still linger around. Those traces remain in the air, in the soil, in several bodies of water – and eventually, in the foods that humanity consumes.

According to Dr. Joseph Mercola, a well-known personality in the US wellness movement and owner and founder of Mercola.com (one of the most-trusted health websites), the ten most common toxic substances that are still prevalent in the environment to this day are the following:

1. Polychlorinated biphenyls, or PCBs, were commonly dumped by factories into nearby bodies of water. Due to their toxicity, PCBs were banned decades ago. However, traces of PCBs can still be found in those bodies of water since the toxic substances do not break down easily even after all those years. Fish that swim in those bodies of water still consume PCBs

unknowingly. As people still eat those fish, they will also ingest PCBs that will contribute to ailments such as cancer and brain defects in newborn babies.

2. Pesticides, while they do kill pests as their name says, are the major contributors of cancer. As farms still use synthetic pesticides such as weed killers, fungi killers, and insect killers; residues of those pesticides still remain in as much as 50 to 90 percent of US farm produce. Furthermore, there are bug sprays used to kill cockroaches and other unwanted insects in homes. Those bug sprays also contain the same carcinogenic substances as farm-focused pesticides. Besides cancer, pesticides also cause Parkinson's disease, miscarriage, nerve damage, birth defects, and getting in the way of nutrient absorption.

3. Fungal toxins not just come in the form of poisonous mushrooms. The most common of those fungal toxins is mould. Mould thrives in moist places such as bathrooms and kitchens; and can even sustain in vulnerable foods such as peanuts, wheat, and corn. One in three people are allergic to this fungal toxin. If left unchecked, mould causes cancer, heart disease, asthma, multiple sclerosis, and diabetes.

4. Phthalates are commonly found in plastic products and are responsible for softening them, making them easier to mold. They can seep into foodstuffs and drinks that are placed inside plastic food containers and plastic bottles. The result of ingesting too much phthalates is hormonal imbalance, since the substances resemble naturally-produced hormones. In children, phthalates can stunt their growth.

5. Volatile organic compounds, or VOCs, are commonly found in several household products such as air fresheners, cleaning fluids, mothballs, and varnishes. VOCs aid in air pollution and cause several sicknesses such as cancer, irritation of eyes and lungs, headaches, dizziness, and impaired memory.

6. Dioxins are some of the pollutants that are produced when something is burned, especially in massive quantities. As they

are released into the air, humans not just breathe in the dioxins. Livestock can also inhale those toxins and settle in their fats even after they are brought to the slaughterhouse to be made into meat. Dioxins cause cancer, stunted growth, reproductive system impairments, skin disorders such as acne, and slight damage to the liver.

7. Asbestos was a popular insulation material, but it was banned in the seventies due to its carcinogenic effects. Traces of asbestos can still be found in old homes that did not have their insulations replaced. Besides cancer, asbestos causes scarring on the lung tissue.

8. Toxic heavy metals such as lead, arsenic, and mercury can still be found in various objects such as cheaply-made toys, preserved wood, antiperspirants, and building materials. Once those metals are inhaled or ingested, they can cause cancer, brain and nerve disorders such as Alzheimer's disease, nausea, lesser amounts of red and white blood cells, and abnormal heartbeats.

9. Chloroform is a common chemical that is used to make other chemicals. It is prevalent in the air, in water, and in food. It can cause cancer, infertility, birth defects, headaches, dizziness, and damage to the liver and kidneys.

10. Chlorine is commonly found in water as it is used to purify it. Whether from the typical drinking water or from a swimming pool, too much of chlorine will cause all sorts of respiratory problems such as sore throat, accumulation of fluid in the lungs, and asthma.

Based on this list, many of those toxins in the environment are brought about by humanity's modern lifestyles. Before they do undue harm to the body, especially the dreaded cancer, they must be flushed out promptly.

Other Sources of Toxins

Besides the ten most common toxic substances, there are also other toxins that can be found in almost everything in the modern world. It is inevitable that one must intake those toxins unknowingly, one way or the other.

The two most popular vices, which are smoking and drinking, are the other major reasons for the body's toxicity. Both alcohol and nicotine have been proven many times by the scientific community to be not just toxic, but also addicting. Those two substances also alter the brain's functions. Other toxic substances include caffeine, empty sugars, and saturated fats. The latter two are especially notorious for being fat fodder since they cannot be processed into needed energy.

Many cosmetics today also contain toxic substances such as VOCs that can be absorbed into the skin. Some cosmetics producers have already taken steps in ridding their beauty products of those toxins.

Taking too many medications all at once can also cause the body to be laced with toxins, since they are not properly eliminated from the body. If the body feels too taxed from a cornucopia of meds, a consultation with the doctor will help.

There are also naturally-occurring toxins that are used by certain plants and animals as defense mechanisms against invaders. Snakes and jellyfish have highly deadly toxins and should not be consumed as food. A Japanese dish called *fugu* uses a type of blowfish that releases toxins which will certainly kill someone who eats an improperly-prepared version of the dish.

Processed foods, especially canned goods, are also a major source of toxins. While those foods contain preservatives that prolong their shelf lives, they unknowingly unleash a world of hurt on one who voraciously eats these. Needless to say, one must balance those foods out with naturally-grown foods.

Chapter 2: Why Must We Detoxify?

Detoxification is not just the simple flushing out of unwanted substances when the body cannot handle expelling them on its own. It is also the purging of impure thoughts in the mind that cause all sorts of decisions to inhale and ingest several toxins, whether knowingly or unknowingly, into the body. To ensure that an individual is rightfully clean in both body and mind, all sorts of unwanted things must be eliminated, especially in the detox diet.

The Body Does It Own Job...

The excretory system does its job of purging waste substances from the body via its two major processes: urination and release of excrement. Urination is obviously handled by the urinary system, while the release of excrement is handled by the lower parts of the digestive system.

The urinary system's main actor is the kidneys. The kidneys filter unwanted stuff such as ammonia, urea, uric acid, and excess salt and water from the blood as well as other bodily fluids. Those unwanted stuff then get to the bladder, which acts as a temporary storage. If the bladder gets full, the stuff gets expelled out of the urethra in the form of urine. Ammonia is a byproduct of the breakdown and usage of protein for the body's energy, while urea and uric acid are less toxic substances that result from the breakdown of ammonia.

The lower parts of the digestive system consist of the liver, the intestines, and the colon. The liver does its job of breaking down foreign substances so that the kidneys can have an easier job filtering them out as urine. The intestines and the colon facilitate the expelling of solid waste substances in the form of feces. The colon, in particular, absorbs trace minerals such as potassium and sends them to the bloodstream before they are included as feces that will be expelled by pooping.

Another natural detoxifier found in the human body is the lymphatic system. The lymphatic system contains lymph nodes that are scattered throughout the body but are interconnected. Those nodes provide the body with immunity, complementing the immune system, by filtering out unwelcome invaders such as bacteria, viruses, old red blood cells, and other toxic substances.

Other parts of the excretory system consist of the lungs and skin. The lungs expel excess water and carbon dioxide when someone breathes out. The skin kicks out excess water, salt, uric acid, and excess trace minerals in the form of sweat.

...But It Is Not Enough in the Modern Age

However, as demonstrated in the previous chapter, there are far too many substances that are deemed toxic in the wrong amounts. With humanity's modern lifestyles, the body does not know what to make of the increasing number of unwelcome invaders in its insides. These usually never get flushed out as urine and feces, but instead accumulate in the body fat.

As the invaders multiply and never get flushed out, they get in the way of the body's usual processes and will cause several problems such as depleted energy levels, unnatural weight gain, and various diseases that target the major body systems.

Another thing that is not helping the body in its natural detoxification process is the busy and hectic schedules people normally have. Because those people have no time to perform even mundane healthy tasks such as drinking adequate water, the body never gets its supply of natural detox assistants. Couple the lack of those assistants with stress and it will be a recipe for disaster.

Therefore, it is important that in this world of toxicity, people must amplify their bodily defenses against all sorts of foreign toxic substances by enhancing the many components of the excretory system such as the kidneys, the liver, the intestines, and the colon. With the contaminants out of the way, the body's natural healing processes also get their groove back. As the major organ systems work hand-in-hand, the benefits that are felt in one particular system will spread towards the other systems.

In short, steeling the body and its functions, especially the excretory functions, is one of the first lines of defense against toxin-induced sicknesses. There will be a marked loss in weight, since the excessive fats as well as the toxins they contain are properly expelled. There will also be renewed liveliness since the bodily functions that have something to do with the intake and processing of energy sources are no longer clogged by invasive toxins.

Why the Mind Is Also Important in Detoxification

The decisions a person makes, no matter how small they are, can contribute to huge consequences. For example, if one decides to commute to a bar, he or she gets all sorts of toxins in the process – airborne impurities from urban roads, food additives from the snacks he or she eats while commuting, nicotine and other chemicals from tobacco smoke generated by smokers inside and outside the bar, and alcohol from the hard drinks he or she consumes while in the bar.

Therefore, it is important that a person must think thoroughly and deeply before settling on a decision that will make him or her take in all those unwanted toxins along the way. Yes, this may turn him or her into a control freak, but there are also decisions that will endow him or her with long-term benefits. Remember, detoxification starts in the mind. The decisions that lead to the unknowing intake of toxins must be sorted out and eliminated from the usual routines first.

Chapter 3: The Crucial Ten Days

There are several forms of detoxification, and they more often than not involve ingesting special liquids and solids, cleansing the colon, foot baths and foot pads, spas and saunas, and fasting. But they also cost money, are always focused on the short-term effects, and may not deliver the detoxification results one desires. The best form of the detox diet must involve getting rid of major sources of toxins, ingesting more of the substances that will greatly assist the body's natural detoxification processes, never integrating any form of starvation or elimination of a major food group from the diet, and clearing the mind of impure thoughts that lead to impure actions. This way, the diet will grant long-term effects of well-being. As a beneficial consequence, this diet will cost little to no money, except for the money to be spent on detoxifying foods and drinks.

The ten days this detox diet contains are important to ensure natural weight loss and general well-being. And even after the diet period ends, some good habits contained in this diet, particularly the continued eating of healthy foods, must still be kept. This is to ensure that the person undergoing this diet will transition into a healthy lifestyle.

Preparing for the Diet

One important thing to do when undergoing this diet, or any other diet for that matter, is to not rush in immediately. A crash diet will have nasty consequences such as abrupt changing of body patterns that lead to all sorts of ailments as well as retention of the weight one lost during the diet routine. Therefore, one must start slow and transition into the diet carefully.

Not rushing in also applies to the chewing of food. The body needs some time to digest the food. Never treat the ten days of the diet like some kind of work deadline.

The usual vice-based sources of toxins, which are tobacco and alcohol, must be eliminated first. While dealing with the withdrawal effects of both of those substances may be difficult, timely help from a doctor who has a specialization in several types of addictions and substance abuse will lessen the difficulty.

In the three days before the actual start of the diet, rid the pantry and fridge of tempting foodstuffs that are loaded with empty calories. These include sweets and most forms of processed foods and fast food. At the same time, steadily increase the intake of fruits and vegetables – *especially organic ones*. As much as possible, turn the veggies into freshly-prepared salads and/or lightly steam them. As for the fruits, eat them raw and/or turn them into natural juices.

Since pesticide residue in fruits and vegetables is inevitable, the use of fruit and vegetable washes must be prioritized.

The intake of caffeine must be slowly and surely reduced to prevent withdrawal symptoms such as headaches. Switching to decaf coffee and low-caffeine teas such as green tea will help, as is the trick of diluting regular coffee and tea in huge amounts of water.

And speaking of water, the time-tested advice of eight to ten glasses of water a day will especially help the detox diet become successful. Drink it throughout the ten days of the diet.

Aromatherapy using essential oils is helpful, as this therapy helps to calm the mind in order for it to prepare for the rigors of the critical ten days.

Finally, before embarking on the detox diet itself, please consult a registered dietician who can recommend the detoxifying foods to be eaten based on your genetic makeup. Furthermore, *do not stop* taking prescribed medicine, as discontinuing medications can have devastating effects on the body. Diets are not meant to be one-man shows, especially if the individual still has to learn much about the intricacies of diet programs like this.

Eat and Drink Them

With the transition phase over, it is time to actually start the detox diet. Here is a comprehensive list of foods and drinks that must be ingested during the ten crucial days of the diet.

1. Organic fruits and vegetables are the main focus of the detox diet. It does not matter what the size or type of fruit or vegetable one will be consuming – as long as it is free of pesticides and synthetic fertilizers and is grown using age-old farming techniques, it certainly counts. Eat a good variety of fruits and vegetables to round out all the necessary nutrients.

2. Brown rice is much healthier compared to the typical white rice. As white rice is a result of the milling process, brown rice retains some nutrients that are usually lost during milling. This type of rice is also a rich source of fiber, which will aid in flushing the toxins out via the intestines and the colon.

3. Herbs are permissible, since they are also plants. Use them to flavor the dishes as well as utilize them for aromatherapy. Herbal teas are also a-OK, since they do not contain caffeine at all. As with fruits and vegetables, herbs must not have traces of anything toxic.

4. Whole-grain products, much like brown rice, do not undergo the nutrient-losing milling process. They are also rich sources of fiber. Whole-grain products include whole wheat bread, bran, and rolled oats.

5. Seaweeds such as kelp and *nori* wrappers used for sushi are also plant-based. They can also be consumed the same way as typical veggies do.

6. Beans such as green peas, chick peas, lentils, kidney beans, and black beans are permitted.

7. One can go nuts with nuts and seeds. Allowable things include almonds, cashews, walnuts, watermelon seeds, pumpkin

seeds, sunflower seeds, and sesame seeds. As a general rule, pick only raw, unsalted nuts and seeds.

8. Coconuts, while they are not actually nuts, are also allowed. There are several coconut-based consumables such as coconut water and coconut oil. One can also eat fresh coconut meat straight from the source.

9. Plant-based oils are encouraged. Olive oil, especially the extra virgin kind, is highly recommended.

10. Round out the protein-based nutrition with plant-based protein sources such as soy. Soy milk and tofu are easily-acquired sources of plant-based protein.

11. All sorts of edible mushrooms are permitted. Portobello and shiitake mushrooms can act as good substitutes for meat.

12. Natural sweeteners such as raw honey and natural maple syrup are permitted.

13. Besides herbs, other natural condiments that are tolerable include apple cider vinegar, sea salt, and mustard.

14. If there is still a desire to eat meat and get adequate protein, go with lean meats such as fish and organic chicken. Eggs are also on the list, as long as they are organic.

Never Eat and Drink Them

Meanwhile, these are the foods and drinks to avoid during the detox diet phase.

1. In general, non-lean types of red meat are off-limits. Canned meat is especially forbidden.

2. All forms of processed foods containing all sorts of additives and preservatives are out of the question. On a related note, artificial sweeteners and processed condiments are also out.

3. Typical white sugar and brown sugar are verboten, as well as high-fructose syrups.

4. Corn must be avoided as it is acid-forming. The acid in question is uric acid. Furthermore, the corn kernels that are indigestible will make bathroom breaks more excruciating.

5. While nuts are OK, peanuts and peanut butter are usually excluded.

6. Milk is normally not allowed, but half a cup of yogurt containing good bacteria per day is an exception to that.

7. Caffeine is another typical forbidden substance.

8. Shortening and margarine are inadmissible.

9. While fish is OK, other seafoods are not.

Other Cleansing Procedures

There are many variations of the detox diet, but the one being presented in this book will not involve complicated doohickeys and specialized food and drinks to amplify the detoxification effect. Here are some things one can also do during the ten days of the diet.

With all the conveniences of Internet-based connectivity, sometimes too much is too much. Dedicate one of the ten days, or even all ten days, to a temporary break from technology. Put away the smartphone or tablet, avoid touching the computer, and never be tempted to go online just about anywhere. Take the time off from technology to visit someplace serene, like a retreat house. This technology break will clear the mind of all sorts of burdening thoughts that may poison one's thinking the same way that bodily toxins do.

Take some time off to scrape the tongue. Tongue scraping is a practice in ayurvedic medicine, or ancient Hindu medicine, where all the impurities built up on the tongue are removed. Tongue scrapers can be bought for cheap at drug store.

Try to write all the stored thoughts and feelings, even negative ones, into a diary or notebook. Releasing all the stored strong emotions to a diary or notebook has a cathartic effect, since keeping those emotions locked away will eventually take the toll on one's health.

Another mind-cleansing procedure one can do during the ten days is meditation. Meditation also helps clear the mind of toxic thoughts that lead to stress, which then slows down the liver's detoxification process. Yoga is especially helpful as a meditation tool. You may also augment your meditation by doing deep breathing exercises or visualizing relaxing images such as watching the sunset at the beach.

Get enough dosages of vitamin C. While the vitamin is better known for boosting immunity, it also helps the body with the production of glutathione. Glutathione may be better known as a skin rejuvenating agent, but it also exists in the liver as a detoxification aid. Citrus fruits are the best-known sources of vitamin C.

Enhance blood circulation, since poor blood circulation will hamper the flushing out of impurities from the blood. Exercise is a guaranteed way to get that blood pumping.

Keep in mind that not all bacteria are bad. Good bacteria mostly reside in the intestines, aiding in digestion and preventing bad bacteria from releasing toxins that can be deployed in the bloodstream. Help the good bacteria by taking probiotic drinks.

Chapter 4: Detoxification Recipes

Breakfast Recipes

Gut-Busting Oatmeal Bowl

Ingredients:

- 1-2 cups oatmeal

- 1-2 cups water or nut milk

- A mixture of fresh berries and fresh fruits, all sliced

Procedure:

1. Prepare the oatmeal as indicated in the packaging.

2. While hot, pour the berries and fruits onto the prepared oatmeal, and mix.

Berry Blast Smoothie

Ingredients:

- 1-2 cups mixed fresh berries
- 1-2 cups protein powder
- 1-2 cups ice cubes

Procedure:

1. Throw all the ingredients into a blender, and hit puree.
2. Serve the smoothie in a tall glass.

Lunch Recipes

Veggie Cavalcade Salad with Tofu

Ingredients:

- 6-8 pieces of any whole vegetable (for greens, an amount of at least five leaves equals one whole piece)

- 1-2 pieces tofu, diced

- 4-5 teaspoons extra virgin olive oil

- 2 teaspoons fresh lemon juice

- 1 teaspoon freshly-chopped herbs of choice

Procedure:

1. Fry the tofu in 2-3 teaspoons olive oil until slightly browned. Set aside.

2. Slice and/or dice the vegetables into reasonably-sized pieces. Leave the greens untouched.

3. Pour all the vegetables and the tofu into a bowl. Mix completely.

4. Combine 2 teaspoons olive oil, the lemon juice, and the herbs to make the dressing.

5. Pour the dressing all over the salad. Mix completely.

Special Omelet Rice

Ingredients:

- 3-5 organic eggs

- Fresh or dried herbs (any variety), to taste

- 2-3 teaspoons extra virgin olive oil

- 1-2 cups cooked brown rice

Procedure:

1. Beat the eggs into a scramble while adding the herbs.

2. Pour the olive oil into a heated pan. Wait until the oil is hot.

3. Pour the egg and herb mixture until the omelet is formed. Turn over to ensure proper cooking.

4. Once the omelet is out of the pan, place the brown rice inside it. Make sure the omelet wraps around the rice.

5. Serve hot with mustard.

Dinner Recipes

The Steamed Medley

Ingredients:

- 1 slice salmon

- 5-10 pieces broccoli and asparagus (can be of any combination)

- 1/4 cup fresh lemon juice

- Fresh or dried herbs (any variety), to taste

Procedure:

1. In a steamer or a rice cooker with a steaming basket, arrange the salmon slice and the broccoli and asparagus pieces so that the steam will be evenly distributed.

2. Sprinkle the salmon and the vegetables with the lemon juice and fresh herbs.

3. Begin steaming the salmon and the vegetables. Seven to ten minutes is enough for the lemon and the herbs to seep into the steamed content.

4. Serve hot.

Glorified Bunch of Small Potatoes

Ingredients:

- 6 ounces small potatoes

- 4 tablespoons extra virgin olive oil

- Any natural condiment of choice

Procedure:

1. Gently simmer the potatoes in water for 5-10 minutes. Drain them off afterwards. Retain the peels beforehand.

2. Heat the olive oil in a roasting tin, but not to burning levels.

3. Roast every side of the potatoes until crisp and golden brown. This will take at most 45 minutes.

4. Serve hot with the condiment of choice.

Snack and Drink Recipes

Veggie Brown Rice Sushi

Ingredients:

- 1 cup cooked brown rice

- 1 *nori* wrapper

- Any sliced or diced vegetable that can fit inside the sushi

Procedure:

1. Mold the brown rice into any shape, whether in a tube form or rolled into a ball. The important thing is that the vegetable must fit inside the sushi.

2. Wrap the *nori* wrapper around the formed brown rice.

3. Repeat steps 1 and 2 for any remaining amounts of vegetables, brown rice, and the *nori* wrapper.

Stretched Herbal Iced Tea

Ingredients:

- 1 bag herbal tea (any kind)
- 1 citrus fruit of choice (e.g. lemon or orange)
- 1 cup briskly-boiled water
- 2-3 cups lukewarm water
- Several ice cubes
- Honey, to taste

Procedure:

1. Depending on the strength of the resultant tea, submerge one teabag into briskly-boiled water.

2. Meanwhile, cut the citrus fruit of choice into slices that can be fit inside a glass.

3. Place the fruit slices into a tall glass that can accommodate at least five cups.

4. Carefully pour both the brewed tea and the lukewarm water into the tall glass at a distance of at least 12 inches from the glass. This is where the "stretched" part comes from, and one must avoid spills during the stretching process.

5. Add some dollops of honey based on the preferred amount of sweetness.

6. Finally, add the ice cubes.

Fruity Shaved Ice

Ingredients:

- 1-2 cups shaved ice

- 1/2-1 cup natural unsweetened fruit juice of any kind

Procedure:

1. Place the shaved ice in either a wide glass or a bowl.

2. Pour the unsweetened fruit juice on top of the shaved ice, and enjoy.

Note: One can replace shaved ice with shaved or crushed frozen fruit.

Chapter 5: Some Friendly Reminders

As with every other diet program on the planet, care, precise planning, patience, and perseverance must be taken to heart when undergoing the detoxification diet. Even in a short period like ten days, many things will happen. To ensure that the detox diet will become a success that will beget many more successes in the realm of the healthy lifestyle, keep the following friendly reminders in mind.

Do Not Starve

Other detox diets recommend taking only the formulas they sell themselves. Indeed, they may contain needed plant-based nourishment needed for detoxification, but the makers of those diets often forget that an imbalanced diet that is lacking in calories will prove detrimental to the body. Not only will the energy levels be depleted, but the metabolism process will also be slowed down. One unpleasant aftereffect is the tendency to eat more, especially unhealthy foods, once the diet period is over. This will make natural weight loss almost unachievable. Even worse, the lack of micronutrients in these other detox diets will lead to malnutrition that is based on micronutrient deficiency, which opens yet another floodgate of diseases. Other nasty effects of other detox crash diets include muscle degeneration, since the muscles have no source of energy to turn to, and an imbalance in blood sugar levels.

Hence, this detox diet espouses the idea that *forced starvation is absolutely prohibited*. Just eat the recommended foods at will and in good, moderated amounts.

Expect to Pee (and Poop and Sweat) a Lot

Since the detox diet enhances the body's natural detox functions, expect one undergoing the diet to pee a lot. Water, in particular, helps in flushing out toxins.

Excessive peeing not just happens when the detox diet goes overboard. Excessive sweating also happens, as well as the resultant excrement being too liquid and nasty-smelling. Peeing, pooping, and sweating too much can lead to dehydration if the amount of fluids being taken is not immediately replenished.

Dehydration is not just the depletion of the body's water, but is also the disrupted balance of fluids and electrolytes that can lead to ailments such as gastrointestinal distress, headaches, fatigue, irritability, skin irritations, circulatory problems, kidney failure, and heat stroke. Death also awaits one who is severely dehydrated.

To counteract dehydration, do not depend on fluids and fluids alone, unlike what some detox diets emphasize. Be well-balanced in both solids and liquids to avoid lost hours as a result of abnormally frequent trips to the bathroom.

Want a Colonic? No Thanks

Another form of the detox therapy involves cleansing the colon and intestines of toxins that may be released into the bloodstream. However, as demonstrated in the third chapter, there are beneficial bacteria that reside in the colon and intestines. If those bacteria are flushed out, the normal digestive process will be hampered, and the bad bacteria will have a good time releasing more toxins since their rivals are gone. The flushing out of good bacteria also results from the detox diet going beyond the recommended ten days.

Another bad effect of colon cleansing is dehydration, for the same reasons demonstrated in the previous section. Trace minerals such as potassium are also lost during the cleansing process, which contributes to dehydration. Other side effects of colon cleansing include nausea and vomiting.

Diet as an End to the Means, Not a Means to the End

People who want the figures of their dreams often forget that dieting is not really meant to immediately shed unwanted pounds. Dieting is truly meant for improved nourishment and nutrition. The notions of shedding that slab or beer belly in preparation for an event like showing off in a bikini should be disposed of. A proper mindset must be established first when doing the detox diet or any other diet for that matter.

As stated before, the detox diet being demonstrated in this book should be a transitional phase to a healthier lifestyle. Thinking in the long term when dieting is certainly better than thinking in the short term. One should remember that dieting must be an end to unhealthy habits and not a means to end that "awful" figure.

Conclusion

Thank you again for purchasing *"Detox Diet Guide: Lose Weight Quickly, Achieve Optimal Health and Feel Energized Through the 10 Day Detox"*!

I hope this book was able to help you to understand the ins and outs of the detox diet and why it is important to achieve a major change in only a short time.

Are you ready for the change? Tony Robbins says in order to create effective change, you need to start by being disgusted with where you are at. Are you disgusted with your health or body? Is it an ABSOLUTE MUST to change...not another moment? You need to feel the pain of where you are at to get the urgency to change and manifest the momentum to take action.

The next step is to consult your doctor or dietician before embarking on such a diet. And once you are given the final OK, you can then consult various more detoxification recipes based on the comprehensive list of allowable foods and drinks in this book. The recipes given in this book is just a starting point.

Finally, if you enjoyed this book, please take the time to share your thoughts and post a review on Amazon. It would be greatly appreciated!

I would love for you to share your experiences, stories and encouragements with me. My email address is

emmarosekindle@gmail.com

In addition, please remember to check out our Facebook page in order to find other resources and upcoming promotions:

https://www.facebook.com/joypublishing

With sincere thanks,

Emma Rose

Emma Rose

Preview Of "Paleo Free Diet Guide for Beginners: Over 50 Paleo Free Diet Recipes for Fast Weight Loss and Optimal Health"

Introduction

I want to thank you and congratulate you for purchasing the book, *"Paleo Free Diet Guide for Beginners: Over 50 Paleo Free Diet Recipes for Optimal Health and Fast Weight Loss"*.

This book contains everything you might need to know when it comes to getting started with the Paleo diet. It is provided in an easily digestible format that allows you to better absorb the information. There are no complicated explanations about how it works! You'll be given what you need straight up so you won't have to waste time trying to understand exactly what the diet is. Whether it's for your overall good health or to lose a few pounds, Paleo can certainly help you with it. To help you get started, we'll do the same and start you off with 50 of the best Paleo recipes that you can slowly but surely shift your everyday menu to.

It's never easy changing a diet. I often fall into self pity when I can no longer have the foods I enjoy. Either I feel sorry for myself or I get rebellious and binge and anything and everything. I always knew the value of eating healthy. I could just never bring myself to do it. It wasn't until I had a miscarriage that I got serious about my health. I have made drastic changes that others just don't understand. But the pay off is the weight I've lost and the better health I'm experiencing.

My hope for you is not to be on another "diet." This isn't a restriction diet like Atkins. The goal is to have a lifestyle change. Lifestyle changes are more sustainable and maintain weight loss long term compared to restriction diets. The change is hard to start but worth it when you commit. The trick is to get the momentum to start.

Thanks again for purchasing this book. I hope you enjoy reading it and eating the recipes from it!

With gratitude,

Emma Rose

Chapter 1 – What Is the Paleo Diet?

The Paleo Diet is known by many names such as the cavemen diet, stone age diet and hunter-gatherer diet, to name a few. The concept behind this diet follows that of the Paleolithic era before the development of agriculture. Essentially, you consume the same foods that the cavemen used to eat. The focus is on eating food closest to its natural, unprocessed state. The cavemen would gather their food from any source available whether it was wild animals, berries, vegetables, or fruits. As a result, they were strong, fit, and healthy for thousands of years.

This type of diet is still very young, less than fifty years only, but more in depth researches and studies are being conducted to increase the information and knowledge on this diet. The results of previous studies conducted on the Paleo diet reveal the improvement of health to the people involved. This is attributed to the fact that no processed foods and additives are included. The Paleo Diet is a diet that works with our genetics – before machinery and processing got involved. Foods that were not available during the Paleolithic time such as dairy products, salt, sugar and grains are not included in the preparation of the Paleo diet.

The modern diet predominately consumed in the Western world is full of refined foods, trans fats, salt and sugar. These ingredients are known to indirectly cause diseases such as hypertension, diabetes, strokes, obesity and other heart problems. The list goes on even further with the increase diagnosis of cancer, Parkinson's, Alzheimer's, depression and infertility. "What an extraordinary achievement for a civilization: to have developed the one diet that reliably makes its people sick!" (Michael Pollen, Food Rules: An Eater's Manual, Penguin Books 2009).

Foods included in the Paleo Diet

- Fruit

- Vegetables

- Lean Meat

- Seafood

- Nuts/Seeds

- Healthy Fats (eg. coconut, avocado, nuts and seeds, olive oil, grass fed butter)

Foods NOT included in the Paleo Diet

- Dairy

- Grain

- Processed Food

Why not grain?

You may be surprised to see that grains are not included in the Paleo Diet. We are accustomed to grains being a part of a balanced diet. However, our bodies are not designed to deal with the nutritional components of grains such as gluten, lectin, and phytates.

Gluten is a protein substance found in wheat, barley and rye. Many people are discovering that their bodies are gluten sensitive and are eliminating gluten from their diet. The most extreme case of gluten sensitivity is Celiac Disease. Individuals with this disease can pick up the minutest trace of gluten and react immediately.

Lectin binds to insulin receptors and can also cause leptin resistance.

Phytates cause minerals to become unavailable during digestion.

Why is dairy a problem?

When purchasing milk, you need to be mindful of the source.

Check out the rest of "Paleo Diet Guide for Beginners: Over 50 Paleo Diet Recipes for Fast Weight Loss and Optimal Health" on Amazon.

Or go to: http://amzn.to/1jIJUFX

Check Out My Other Books

Below you'll find some of my other books also available on Amazon and Kindle. Search for these titles on the Amazon website to find them.

Paleo Free Diet Guide for Beginners: Over 50 Paleo Free Recipes for Optimal Health & Fast Weight Loss

Paleo Desserts: Satisfy Your Sweet Tooth With Over 100 Quick & Easy Paleo Dessert Recipes & Paleo Baking Recipes

Raw Food Diet Guide: Lose Weight Quickly, Achieve Optimal Health & Feel Energized with the Raw Food Diet & Raw Food Recipes

Clean Eating Guide: Lose Weight Quickly, Achieve Optimal Health & Feel Energized with Clean Eating For Busy Families & Clean Eating Recipes

Alkaline Diet Guide: Lose Weight Quickly, Achieve Optimal Health & Feel Energized with the Alkaline Diet & Alkaline Recipes

Coconut Flour Recipes for Optimal Health & Quick Weight Loss: Gluten Free Recipes for Celiac Disease, Gluten Sensitivities & Paleo Free Diets

Almond Flour Recipes for Optimal Health & Quick Weight Loss: Gluten Free Recipes for Celiac Disease, Gluten Sensitivities & Paleo Free Diets

Wheat Free Diet for Beginners: Lose Weight Quickly, Achieve Optimal Health & Feel Energized with Gluten Free Recipes for Celiac Disease, Gluten Sensitivities & Paleo Free Diets

Detox Diet Guide: Lose Weight Quickly, Achieve Optimal Health & Feel Energized Through the 10 Day Detox

Sugar Detox Guide for Beginners: Lose Weight Quickly, Achieve Optimal Health, Feel Energized & Eliminate Sugar Cravings Naturally

Ketogenic Diet Guide for Beginners: How to Achieve Rapid Weight Loss, Optimal Health & Unstoppable Energy with Ketogenic Diet Recipes

Anti Inflammatory Diet for Beginners: Lose Weight Fast, Optimize Health, Slow Aging, Fight Inflammation, Conquer Pain & Increase Energy with the Anti Inflammation Diet Recipes

One Last Thing...

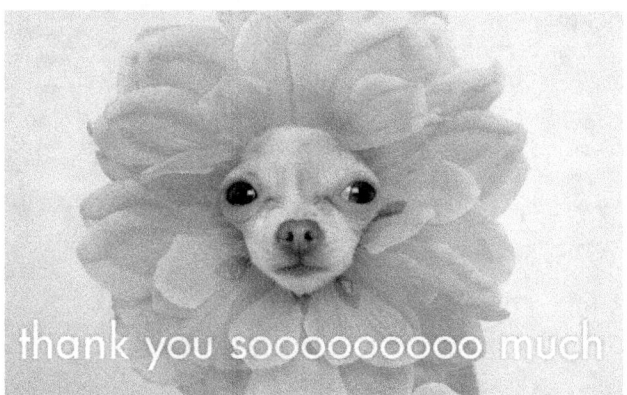

Source: Wikipedia

If you believe that this book is worth sharing, would you please take the time to let others know how it affected your life? If it turns out to make a difference in the lives of others, they will be forever grateful to you, as will I.